Familiarity with ultrasound and its application in medicine

Mahdi Kolahdouz Ghouchani

Farshid Aramjoo

ISBN:9798321192092

Contents

Introduction -- 2

History of ultrasound from the beginning ---------------------- 3

Important points in buying an ultrasound machine --------- 20

Application of sonotherapy --------------------------------------- 27

What is portable ultrasound? ------------------------------------- 30

Types of pregnancy ultrasound ---------------------------------- 40

Is ultrasound painful? -- 46

Application of ultrasound in children and babies ------------ 53

Veterinary ultrasound device applications ---------------------- 70

Resources --- 76

Introduction

This book is written in a simple and understandable tone to familiarize the general public with ultrasound.

With the development of medical science, ultrasound has made many changes and plays a significant role in the diagnosis and treatment of diseases. The development of medicine and the progress of treatment methods are due to these changes in ultrasound. Unfortunately, the general public, with a misunderstanding of the benefits and harms of ultrasound, have a series of wrong beliefs and expectations, which we have tried to introduce in this book and remove the ambiguities.

It is hoped that by reading this book, the science and knowledge of different societies about ultrasound will increase and we will see the progress of ultrasound and its methods as quickly as possible, as well as the progress of medical science.

History of ultrasound from the beginning

The origin of ultrasound can be found in ancient Greece. You must have heard of Pythagoras, when Pythagoras was solving puzzles related to right triangles, he invented a device called a sonometer, which was used to study musical sounds.

In 1790, Lazzaro Spallanzani used waves to navigate bats flying in the dark and proved that bats use light and sound to navigate.

The role of piezoelectricity in the discovery of ultrasound

In 1880, Galton built a device capable of producing sound waves with a frequency of 40 Hz. Then a person named Pierre Curie together with his brother discovered a device called piezoelectric in 1877. Many physicists associate the invention of ultrasound with the discovery of piezoelectricity. Of course, 35 years after this incident, ultrasound was created by a famous professor and physicist named Paul Langevin.

The invention of X-rays

In 1895, William Conrad Roentgen succeeded in discovering X-rays. But the interesting point in the history of ultrasound is that it was only after the sinking of the Titanic in 1912 that people became interested in discovering sunken objects under the sea.

Following this incident, Constantin Chilovsky proposed the idea of ultrasonic detection system. This idea, which was proposed at the same time as the First World War, was highly regarded by French government officials. As a result, the French government asked Paul Langevin, who happened to be Pierre Curie's assistant, to build this device so that they could identify enemy submarines during the war.

Sonar (sound and range navigation)

Although Langevin did not succeed in building such a device, these efforts led to the recognition of the basis of sonar detection, which was developed during World War II. This sonar device was used to identify underwater objects such as icebergs. It wasn't until the mid-1930s that most ocean liners had some form of sonar.

Ultrasound and medicine

In the 1920s and 1930s, ultrasound was used as a physical therapy tool for members of European football teams. It was also used to treat cancers along with radiation therapy.

In the 1940s, ultrasound was used as a pain reliever for all diseases, from arthritis pain to stomach ulcers, even for eczema and hemorrhoids. But Karl Dussik, a neurologist and psychiatrist in Austria, was the first to use ultrasound to diagnose diseases.

Following this incident, George Ludwig, who worked at the US Naval Research Institute, used ultrasound to diagnose gallstones. His pioneering research on the interactions between ultrasound waves and animal tissues laid the foundation for subsequent successes in ultrasound.

B mode scanner

In 1949, Douglas Howry, a radiologist at the University of Colorado working in his basement, was able to produce a pulse echo ultrasound scanner using 2.5 MHz. John Reid and John Wild were other people who contributed to the history of sonography and in 1950 they developed a linear B-mode instrument for breast tumors. In 1951, Joseph Holmes and

Harvey were able to build the first two-dimensional B-mode linear combination scanner.

Initially, the scanning equipment was very large, so that the first B-scanner filled a 3.5 x 3.5 room. But it was the invention of the transistor and finally the integration of circuits that made the manufacturing equipment smaller.

Wolf D. Keidel was the first to use ultrasound on the heart. Then in 1953, when a physicist from Lund University named Hellmuth Hertz met by chance with Inge Edler, who was a cardiologist, the beginning of echocardiography was formed.

Pregnancy ultrasound

The late 1960s and early 1970s were known as the Sonic Boom, and it was during this period that 2D echo was introduced by Klaus Bom. Later, with the help of his engineering team, Don Baker developed color Doppler and two-dimensional scanning.

Finally, ultrasound, which is used for pregnancy today, came into existence in the early 1980s. In 1990, ultrasound was accompanied by three-dimensional and even four-dimensional images. As a result, the patient could also see what the doctor diagnosed. A decade later, the basis for the construction of Doppler ultrasound was created on this basis.

It was in 1973 that the profession of sonography was established through training in the United States. As a result, training for it was needed, and after several years of forming a committee to write the requirements document, the Joint Review Committee on Training in Medical Sonography was finally established in 1979.

What is ultrasound imaging?

Ultrasound is safe and painless and produces images of the inside of the body using sound waves. This imaging involves the use of a small transducer (probe) and gel that is placed directly on the skin.

High-frequency sound waves are transmitted from the probe through the gel to the body. Ultrasound examinations do not use harmful radiation (as used in X-rays), so they are not dangerous for the patient.

Types of ultrasound: (general classification)

There are basically seven different methods, but the basic process is the same. The different types of methods are:

1- Transvaginal ultrasound: They are used to produce ultrasound images inside the vagina, and transvaginal ultrasound is often used during early pregnancy.

2- Conventional ultrasound: an examination that uses a transducer and takes place in different areas of the body such as the abdomen to produce two-dimensional images of the developing fetus.

3- Specialized ultrasound: This examination is similar to a normal ultrasound, but this type of examination targets a suspected problem and more complex equipment is used.

4- Color Doppler imaging: This imaging method measures slight changes in the frequency of ultrasound waves, because they image moving objects such as blood cells.

5- 3D ultrasound: using pre-designed special probes and specialized software, for example, to produce 3D images of the developing fetus.

6- 4D or 3D dynamic ultrasound: It is designed using specially designed scanners and is used, for example, to look at the face and movements of the child before delivery.

What are some common uses of ultrasound?

Ultrasound can help diagnose diseases by detecting and evaluating body injuries in different conditions.

Also to help doctors from symptoms such as:

- the pain
- Swelling
- Infection

This type of imaging is a useful method for examining many internal organs of the body, some of the more important ones include:

- Heart and blood vessels, including the abdominal aorta and its main branches
- Liver
- Gallbladder
- Spleen
- Pancreas
- kidneys

Bladder (such as diagnosing varicocele in men

- Uterus, ovaries and pregnancy ultrasound

- eyes
- Thyroid and parathyroid glands
- Scrotum (testicles)
- Infant brain
- Neonatal pelvis
- Spine in babies
- Soft tissue and breast
- Elastography of the liver (fibroscan) and other areas
- Elastography of breast masses

What is color doppler ultrasound and what are its uses?

Color Doppler ultrasound is one of the main methods for diagnosing deep vein thrombosis (DVT). A disease in which blood clots get stuck in the blood vessels, especially in the legs. This disease can cause many problems, including the accumulation of blood clots in the lungs and endanger the patient's life. Therefore, color Doppler ultrasound is necessary for these patients if symptoms are observed. In addition, color doppler ultrasound in pregnant women is also performed under special conditions, which will be explained below.

Why is color Doppler ultrasound performed?

If you feel any of the symptoms of DVT syndrome, such as swelling, coldness, or pain in the legs, your doctor will use a color Doppler ultrasound to examine your blood vessels in order to detect possible blood clots. In other cases, the doctor may prescribe a Doppler ultrasound test if you have the following symptoms:

- feeling exhausted

- Shortness of breath

- Abdominal swelling or swelling in the leg or ankle

- Doctors usually recommend Color Doppler ultrasound to the following patients

- Possible damage to blood vessels as a result of physical injuries

- He has recently been treated for cardiovascular disorders.

- A patient who has recently had a stroke or heart attack

Parts of the produced images that show slow blood flow indicate blockage of blood vessels in that area of the body. In addition to finding blood clots, color Doppler ultrasound may be used in the following cases:

- Checking the blood flow in the veins, vessels and heart

- Check narrowed and blocked veins

- Checking the amount of blood supply in the target area after treatment

- Observation of thinning and swelling of a part of the vessel wall, which is called an aneurysm.

- Application of color doppler ultrasound in the abdominal area in order to detect the following cases

- Blood circulation problems in organs such as kidney, liver, pancreas and spleen

- Abdominal aortic aneurysm

- Doppler ultrasound may also be used to check the baby's blood flow during the mother's pregnancy.

Advantages of using color Doppler ultrasound

- Creating clear color images of blood circulation in the blood vessels of different organs

- Rapid identification of blood vessels, vessel valves and blood circulation disorders in them

- Evaluation of the direction and intensity of blood circulation in blood vessels

- Color Doppler ultrasound in pregnancy

- Women need to undergo ultrasound at least three to four times during pregnancy and at different times to ensure the health of the fetus. NT ultrasound, screening, color doppler, anomaly, etc. are different types of ultrasound that are performed during pregnancy.

Color Doppler ultrasound in pregnant women is usually recommended in the following cases:

- Low fetal growth rate

- History of abortion

- History of giving birth to a child with organ or microorganism defects

- Excessively low or high body mass index (BMI) in the mother

- High blood pressure or diabetes in the mother

• Smoking during pregnancy

• Types of color doppler ultrasound in pregnancy

Color Doppler ultrasound of pregnancy has different types which are introduced below.

• Color Doppler vaginal ultrasound

This ultrasound is done to detect an ectopic pregnancy.

Advantages of using color Doppler ultrasound

• Creating clear color images of blood circulation in the blood vessels of different organs

• Rapid identification of blood vessels, vessel valves and blood circulation disorders in them

• Evaluation of the direction and intensity of blood circulation in blood vessels

• Color Doppler ultrasound in pregnancy

• Women need to undergo ultrasound at least three to four times during pregnancy and at different times to ensure the health of the fetus. NT ultrasound, screening, color doppler, anomaly, etc. are different types of ultrasound that are performed during pregnancy.

Color Doppler ultrasound in pregnant women is usually recommended in the following cases:

• Low fetal growth rate

• History of abortion

- History of giving birth to a child with organ or microorganism defects

- Excessively low or high body mass index (BMI) in the mother

- High blood pressure or diabetes in the mother

- Smoking during pregnancy

- Types of color doppler ultrasound in pregnancy

Color Doppler ultrasound of pregnancy has different types which are introduced below.

- **Color Doppler vaginal ultrasound**

This ultrasound is done to detect an ectopic pregnancy.

Color Doppler sonography of the uterine artery

This type of ultrasound is recommended for women who have a high probability of preeclampsia. In this disorder, the mother may have convulsions and death due to high systolic blood pressure. This disorder also harms the fetus.

Doppler ultrasound of the umbilical artery

This ultrasound is usually performed in women who are pregnant with twins or whose fetuses grow slowly. This ultrasound evaluates the blood flow in the fetus through the umbilical cord to ensure the health of the fetus and sufficient blood supply to various organs, including the brain and heart of the fetus.

How to prepare for color doppler ultrasound?

It is usually necessary to wear comfortable and loose clothes on the day of the test to get better results from color Doppler ultrasound. However, you may be asked to change your clothes to a special medical gown at the ultrasound center. In addition, on the day of imaging, preferably avoid using ornaments and jewelry and keep all metal objects away from you. If color Doppler ultrasound is performed to diagnose DVT, you do not need to do anything else.

How is color doppler ultrasound done?

To do a color Doppler ultrasound, you usually lie on your back on a special ultrasound bed. Then the sonographer rubs a special gel on the desired area. This gel helps to move the special ultrasound series more easily and remove the air between the series and the skin of the body in order to get better results. Then the sonographer will place the special ultrasound series on your skin and move it slowly over the desired area.

Using a special ultrasound series that has a shape similar to a microphone, sound waves hit the tissues of the desired area for imaging. These waves pass through the surface of blood cells such as red blood cells and other body organs and then return to the ultrasound machine. During the Doppler ultrasound, you may feel a little pressure in the imaging area, which is completely normal and painless.

The imaging results are quickly processed and prepared by the computer and referred to the doctor in order to interpret the color Doppler ultrasound results. This test is completely safe and painless and does not use dangerous radiation, so it can be performed during pregnancy and does not cause any harm to the fetus.

Interpretation of color Doppler ultrasound results

The results of color doppler ultrasound of blood vessels help doctors to check the health of veins and blood vessels. Normal results show that the blood vessels do not have any blockage or narrowing. If the sonographer notices any of the following abnormalities, he will include it in his report to the doctor:

• Presence of blood clots

• Obstruction in blood vessels and capillaries

• Narrowing of a vessel

• Spasm of one of the coronary arteries of the heart as a result of stress

Some factors may cause deviations and errors in color Doppler ultrasound results. These factors include:

• Obesity

• Irregular heartbeat

• Cardiovascular diseases

• Smoking before imaging

• Usually, the ultrasound technician does not discuss the Doppler ultrasound results with the patient and sends these results directly to the doctor for interpretation. Your doctor is responsible for interpreting the results of the vascular Doppler ultrasound and talking to you about any possible problems with your blood vessels.

What is meant by four-dimensional ultrasound?

The ultrasounds that can be seen in black and white in the photo are two-dimensional ultrasounds, but three-dimensional and four-dimensional ultrasounds are very similar to each other. Four-dimensional ultrasound is the same as moving three-dimensional. 3D is a color image, and the next four is a color film. In addition to seeing the face and movements of the fetus, you can see the reactions of the fetus during a certain time. For example, the mother can make movements such as hiccups, yawns, and sucking her baby's thumb. to see

Advantages of four-dimensional ultrasound

In fact, the main purpose of doing this ultrasound is to see the fetus more closely, and it can increase maternal feelings, and some mothers who experience despair or despair during pregnancy become more motivated and, for example, improve their nutrition. Or they take more care of their fetus and after they are sure of his health, they do their activities with less stress.

How to perform four-dimensional ultrasound

1. At first, the person is asked to undress his stomach area and lie on the bed.

2. Then the sonographer smears the person's abdomen with a special gel. This is to capture sound waves from the target area.

3. The sonographer moves the transducer (a special tool for ultrasound) inside the abdomen in a rotational manner.

4. These waves are transferred to the monitor and become visible images.

5. If the fetus moves or has a smile-like expression, it can be seen in the images.

6. Images obtained from four-dimensional ultrasound can be recorded and archived.

Important recommendations in four-dimensional ultrasound

Four-dimensional ultrasound is not mandatory for all people, and it should be used if the doctor decides to do it.

The information obtained from this ultrasound is accurate and does not cause any harm to the mother or the fetus.

Since the ultrasound device must be standard, you must visit a center that complies with this.

Ultrasound should be used when needed, otherwise it has harm to the fetus and mother. (Dr. Zohra Mohammadzadeh)

Ultrasound device components:

Each ultrasound device consists of three main parts:

• Monitor that is responsible for displaying images and information.

• Power, which is the device's power source.

• Probe device, the most used types of which are curved or convex, flat or linear, trans-vaginal and phase array.

What features should an ultrasound machine have?

• The high accuracy of the device when imaging in any working mode and the durability of its quality.

• Uniformity and no distortion of the observed and printed image in different imaging modes.

• Absence of noise from city electricity frequency.

• The well-known brand of the device and the history and credibility of the company providing it.

In order to obtain a suitable and efficient image, in addition to the mentioned features, the skill of the operator is also very important. The doctor or the technician who performs the ultrasound operation must be able to adjust the location of the probe and its proper angle to obtain an efficient image.

Although the quality of the images obtained from the ultrasound machine is not comparable with the images of other imaging equipment such as MRI, but this machine is one of the most popular imaging equipment. This can be for the following reasons:

• This product is less expensive than other equipment and its use is less complicated.

• When using this device, dangerous waves such as X-rays or gamma are not used, and it does not require a special ionizing substance, so it is less risky for the patient and the operator.

• A unique feature of this type of imaging is obtaining images in real time. This feature can be very useful especially during surgeries.

• This method is non-invasive and painless in most cases. Therefore, it does not cause discomfort to the patient.

Important points in buying an ultrasound machine:

• The most important thing to consider when choosing the right ultrasound device is the type of activity of the center and the use of the device. The doctor's field of activity is influential in the selection of software and equipment.

• Predicting the number of patients and the amount of use of the device is another point that can help in buying the right device.

• Checking the quality of the device is an important issue that should be considered in choosing the device. It is better to check the quality of images in different modes and their uniformity.

• The device must be updatable and it must be possible to upgrade it in terms of hardware and software.

Ease of use of the device, the volume of the device to store images, the cost of the consumables of the device and the support of the seller's company are among other things that should be considered when choosing an ultrasound device.

Important points in maintaining and cleaning the ultrasound machine:

• The most important point in the maintenance of the ultrasound machine is the maintenance and protection of the probe of the machine. Ultrasound device probes are very sensitive to impact, and if hit, there was a possibility of breaking or damaging the piezoelectric crystals.

• Alcoholic solutions should not be used continuously to clean the device probe. The use of probe covers eliminates the need for repeated sterilization with disinfectant solutions. To clean the probe, it is better to use soft and wet wipes and solutions approved by the manufacturer. Parts of the probe that enter the body must be disinfected before and after each use, even if a sterile cover is used.

• A soft cloth and sometimes an ammonia-based solution are usually used to clean the device monitor. It is better not to use paper towels because it can scratch the surface of the monitor.

• The external parts of the device can be cleaned with a soft cloth and a mild mixture of soap and water.

• Device wires and probes are among the things that should be separated and arranged so as not to cause damage to different parts of the device.

Types of ultrasound probes and their uses

An ultrasound probe is a tool that can create a reflection of tissues and organs by receiving sound and transmitting its reflection. This device, which is generally electronic or in some cases mechanical, actually converts one type of energy into another. The transducer or probe is an essential part of the ultrasound machine. The probe emits ultrasound waves into the body and receives the reflection of the generated waves, and by transferring them to the computer, it finally leads to the creation of an image.

Classification of ultrasound probes

There are different categories for the types of ultrasound probes that work based on ultrasound waves.

Heart probe: Heart probe is used in echocardiography test. In some cases, due to the low frequency, these probes can also be used for abdominal studies.

Vascular probe: A vascular probe is commonly used to image the carotid arteries and veins, including those in the legs. The probe is also used for thyroid imaging, guided injections, and in some cases, when the frequency is high enough, for breast exams. The important point here is that performing the test with this probe in breast examinations should not replace mammography, but the two should be used together.

Abdominal probes: Abdominal probes are used to image organs such as kidney, liver, spleen and stomach. Generally, gynecology/obstetric examinations are done with abdominal transducers.

Vaginal probes: Transvaginal probes are used to conduct studies of women in different stages of pregnancy by entering the vagina of women.

Endorectal probes: Endorectal probes are usually used to check for rectal (anal) cancer, and urologists usually use this type of probe.

Finally, there is the TEE echocardiography transducer, which is passed through the esophagus and is used to evaluate heart studies using the echo transducer. An echo transducer creates sound waves for TEE. This probe is connected to a very narrow tube and goes through my mouth down my throat and into my esophagus. Because the esophagus is so close to the upper chambers of the heart, it creates clear images of the heart's structures and valves.

Types of ultrasound probes and their uses

Ultrasound probes come in different shapes and sizes because the function of each one is different and specific to the same probe. The probes can be placed on the surface of the body or enter the patient's body. Probes are also classified based on the three features of piezoelectric crystal arrangement, printer and frequency. In the following article, three of the most commonly used ultrasound probes were introduced and analyzed:

linear probe

In this series of probes, the positioning of the piezoelectric crystal is linear. The shape of the field of this probe is rectangular. The linear probe creates high-quality and high-resolution images of organs close to the body surface (skin). This makes the probe suitable for vascular imaging and some complex procedures such as central line determination. Its small printer, frequency and application of linear probes depend on whether the imaging is 2D or 3D.

The linear probe for 2D imaging has a wide footprint with a center frequency of 2.5-12 MHz. This probe can be used for various imaging such as vascular tests, angiogenesis of blood vessels, breast, thyroid and tendons, laparoscopy, during surgery, measuring the thickness of body fat and muscles for daily care and checks. Locomotive syndrome and... used.

The linear probe for 3D imaging has a wide range and its central frequency is 7.5-11 MHz. This probe is suitable for breast, thyroid and carotid artery imaging.

Curved probe or canox

In this series of probes, the arrangement of piezoelectric crystals is curved. Also, the shape of the field in Canox probes is curved and wedge-shaped. These models of probes are suitable for depth imaging, although the resolution of the images decreases as the imaging depth increases. Like linear probes, in Canox probes, its small printer, frequency and type of probe application depends on whether it is 2D or 3D imaging.

Canox probe for 2D imaging has wide range and center frequency of 2.5-7.5 MHz. This probe is used for transversal, abdominal imaging and organ detection.

Canox probe has a wide field of view for 3D imaging and its central frequency is 3.5-6.5 MHz. This probe can be used for abdominal studies. In addition to the Canox probe, there is also a smaller probe called the Microcanox, which is used for babies and children.

Fuzzy array probe

These probes have a small printer and their frequency is low in the range of 2-7.5 MHz. The field of view in these probes is narrow, but this matter is very dependent on the frequency. In addition, the shape of the field is triangular (triangular) and the resolution of their images is weak near the field. Phased array probes are usually used in cardiac, abdominal and brain tests.

Other types of ultrasound probes

Pencil probes, which are also called CW Doppler probes, are used to measure blood flow and sound speed in blood. These probes have a small printer that has a low frequency of 2-8 MHz.

Another type of probes are endocavity probes that provide the chance of internal imaging. These probes are designed according to the conditions of placement in body cavities. Endocrine probes include endovaginal, endorectal and cavity imaging probes. In general, the printer of these probes is small and has different frequencies in the range of 3.5-11.5 MHz.

In addition, there are transesophageal TEE probes, which, like endocrine probes, have a small printer and are used for internal tests. This probe enters the patient's body through the esophagus and is usually used in cardiology (heart examination) in order to obtain better heart images. The frequency of these probes is in the middle range, between 3-10 MHz. In addition, some probes are also designed for surgical applications such as laparoscopy.

What is sonotherapy and what are its uses?

Sonotherapy is the treatment of pain and other problems using ultrasound waves. Ultrasound waves are mechanical waves and therefore these mechanical vibrations in the tissue cause the production of heat, and it is this heat that can be soothing. Emerging ultrasound-stimulated treatments can provide an alternative to these treatments with increased efficacy, greater penetration depth, and reduced side effects. Sonodynamic therapy can be used to treat cancers and other diseases such as atherosclerosis, reducing the risk associated with other treatment strategies; Because it induces cytotoxic effects only in the case of external stimulation by ultrasound and only in the cancerous area, unlike systemic administration. Ultrasound with variable and low frequencies is used in physiotherapy to reduce inflammation and pain. It can also be used for heat. For example, ultrasound waves are used to burn tumors and in some cases to stimulate neurons in neurological diseases.

Application of sonotherapy

Thermal application of sonotherapy

With the absorption of ultrasound waves by the body, part of its energy is converted into heat. Local heat from the absorption of ultrasound waves accelerates healing. It increases the elasticity of collagen (elastic protein). It increases the elasticity of scars and improves them. If the scar is attached to the underlying tissues, it causes them to be released. The heat produced by ultrasound waves is different from the heat produced by heating.

Mechanical micromassage

- During the compression and expansion of the environment, ultrasonic longitudinal waves affect the tissue and cause the movement of interstitial water and thus reduce swelling (accumulation of interstitial water as a result of hitting a place).

- Treatment of fresh injury and swelling: Fresh injury is usually associated with swelling. Ultrasound is used in many cases to destroy excretory substances due to impact and reduce the risk of tissue sticking together.

- Treatment of old or chronic swelling: ultrasound sonotherapy breaks the adhesions that may be formed between adjacent structures.

Treatment of sexual problems

Half of men between the ages of 40 and 70 have erectile dysfunction or impotence due to physical or psychological reasons. Normally, the brain sends signals to the nerves to increase blood flow to the penis and cause an erection.

Using the sonotherapy method, we can treat semi-deep tissues such as joints, tendons, ligaments, muscles, etc. Also, this method is widely used in bone fracture repair. One of the cases where sonotherapy is used as a specific treatment is the treatment of facial muscle paralysis. In this disease, due to the fact that the use of usual physiotherapy methods cause the evaporation of eye water, it is possible to easily create heat only at the desired depth by using sonotherapy.

Sonotherapy performance

In general, ultrasound waves are transmitted to the tissue in two ways:

1. Direct contact in which gel is used between the tissue and the transducer.

2. Indirect treatment which is usually underwater treatment and is usually used for surfaces with uncertain shapes such as toes.

Also, there are two ways to move Head therapy:

1. Dynamic method in which we move the probe regularly. This method has the advantage that it does not cause point expansion of the arteries. We place the tissue in a point of the radiation field that has a very high intensity, and we move the treatment head in circular or translational movements with slow movements.

2. Static method, in this method the probe is stationary and emits waves with high intensity to the desired area.

Complications of sonotherapy

• Create a hole or cavitation

One of the factors that reduce the energy of ultrasound waves when passing through body tissues is the creation of cavities or cavitation. All solutions contain a significant amount of invisible gas bubbles, and the large amplitude of ultrasound wave oscillations inside the solutions can cause biological changes on the tissues (tear in the cell wall and disintegration of large molecules).

• Burns

If the waves are used continuously and in one place without rotation, it will cause a burn in the tissue and the waves must be moved.

• Chromosomal rupture

Long-term use of ultrasound waves with very high intensity shows rupture in the DNA strand.

What is portable ultrasound?

Portable ultrasound has a function like other fixed ultrasound devices available in medical centers and clinics, and it helps to observe the internal organs of the body and identify the disease by using sound waves and frequencies. In fact, portable ultrasound is smaller than the ultrasound machines that are located in medical centers. The small size of this device makes it easy to carry and move.

Portable ultrasound consists of a section called ultrasound probe, which emits all sound waves. These waves hit the body organs and after returning, they will show the image of the desired organ on the screen.

After the sonographer receives the images of the internal organs of the body, it transmits them to the processor. The processor analyzes all the images and finally the final image is shown on the screen. Based on this image, information about the target organ or the patient's condition will be recorded.

With a simple review, you can see that this device is no different from other ultrasound devices. Because of its small size and portability, it even has advantages over other devices.

Applications of portable ultrasound

Portable ultrasound does not have any restrictions for performing ultrasound services and observing different parts of the internal organs of the body. As a result, it can be used like normal ultrasounds. In the following, we will tell you some of the uses of this device:

• Analysis of the state of body organs

The most important organs that are examined and analyzed in ultrasound are organs such as the liver and heart. Identification of blockages and clogging in heart vessels is done by ultrasound devices. On the other hand, diseases related to the liver such as; Fatty liver, accumulation of toxins in the liver, and similar cases can also be easily diagnosed with the help of liver ultrasound.

Therefore, in many cases, the doctor can quickly check the condition of the body organs with portable ultrasound, without the need for the patient to go to hospitals and clinics.

• Checking the health of the organs

Another important use of portable ultrasound is that it can examine all the organs of the body in terms of disease, pain, inflammation and infection and provide you with a complete checkup. Especially the pains whose source is internal and cannot be easily detected are identified with the help of this device.

• Observe the state of the gallbladder and kidneys

If the patient feels severe pain in his kidney or excessive secretion of bile causes serious symptoms in the body, the doctor cannot easily diagnose the disease until he sees the results of your ultrasound. For this reason, this device is needed to identify toxins, kidney stones, and similar cases.

If the patient has severe pain, it is very difficult to go to medical centers and perform ultrasound. In this case, the doctor can improve the speed of diagnosis and treatment by using portable ultrasound.

• Observing the general condition of the liver and intestines

Portable ultrasound can also be used to diagnose some general problems in the liver and intestines. But usually, endoscopy should be used in accurate diagnosis of liver and intestinal problems. Using a disposable endoscope is a safe method for diagnosing internal diseases; Because it is completely sterile and safe.

• Examining the baby's health and diagnosing women's diseases

Many women need ultrasound due to the occurrence of certain diseases related to their uterus and ovaries. One of the most important uses of portable ultrasound is that it can even provide the mother with detailed information about the state of the fetus and its health.

Also, if you suffer from diseases such as polycystic ovaries, urinary infections or problems related to the uterus and ovaries, the doctor can easily diagnose the presence of these diseases using a vaginal ultrasound device and start treatment.

• Checking the health of newborns

Ultrasound emits waves to view the internal organs of the body. These waves are not harmful to an adult. They are also completely safe for a baby or child. As a result, they can also be used to identify the internal state of the baby's body. Problems that occur in the heart and brain of babies can be easily diagnosed with the help of portable ultrasound.

• Examination of men's diseases

In addition to women's diseases, there are many diseases that men also need ultrasound because of them. For example, diseases such as varicocele or pain in the testicles and penis can indicate certain diseases that can only be diagnosed by ultrasound. Doctors can easily diagnose these types of diseases by using portable ultrasound as well as fixed ultrasound devices.

Portable ultrasound is used in many other cases. Facial ultrasound for injecting gel and Botox is another application of these devices that can greatly reduce the possibility of medical errors.

How to work with portable ultrasound

Due to its small size and portability, this device has a simple operation, and how to work with it is very convenient and similar to a furnished ultrasound machine.

- Turn on the device

First, the patient should lie on a flat surface and remove all metal objects such as jewelry or bracelets from his body. Then the doctor should turn on the device.

- Pouring special gel

In the next step, a special gel should be poured on the desired organ for ultrasound and completely cover the desired part. This gel helps the device absorb the sound waves that it sends to the internal organs of the body exactly at the desired point and the image waves that come back from it are clearer.

- Placing the transducer on the body

Depending on the location of the test, if needed, the patient should drink and drink liquids before the ultrasound to keep his bladder full. The fullness of the bladder is very important, especially in cases where the health of the bladder and penis is evaluated by the device.

Finally, after taking the necessary images of the target organ at the necessary angles, the portable ultrasound work is finished.

Imaging process with portable ultrasound

The imaging process with portable ultrasound is as follows:

1. Portable ultrasound has a handle or transducer on which a part is placed that emits sound waves. When the sound waves leave the series on the device's transducer, they enter the body with the help of a special gel that is on the surface of the skin, and in this way, they hit the target organ.

2. After impact, these sound waves are reflected from the surface of the body and their reflection hits the transducer and finally turns into image waves that are transferred to the display screen through the processor.

3. The image that is sent to the screen is printed with the help of printer devices or even has the ability to be transferred to other software and provides the possibility of receiving different outputs for the operator or doctor. This image is very accurate and has no difference with the image of fixed ultrasound devices.

Types of portable ultrasound

Portable ultrasound, like fixed ultrasound devices, has not entered the market in just one form and application, but has different types. In the following, we describe some types of portable ultrasound:

Portable laptop ultrasound

There is a type of portable ultrasound devices called laptop devices.

Portable laptop ultrasound features:

- As their name suggests, these devices are very similar to laptops and can be used to examine and analyze all body organs.

- To use this type of device, a battery is used and it weighs almost as much as other portable ultrasound devices.

- This device is able to show the reflection of the images from the converter at a very high speed on the screen. Also, the image display is very clear and of high quality.

Ultrasound with a separate monitor

Another type of portable ultrasound devices are devices that are similar to laptop ultrasound devices in terms of functionality and function, and are actually called portable systems.

Features of ultrasound with a separate monitor:

- The difference of this type of device is that usually the display screen is separate from the rest of the device components. First, to use this type of ultrasound device, it must be connected to a suitable screen.

- These devices are lighter than laptop portable ultrasound devices.

Mobile portable ultrasound

Another type of portable ultrasound device is mobile ultrasound.

Features of portable mobile ultrasound:

- As it is clear from the name of these devices, they have a very small size and their weight is also very low. These devices are also called pocket ultrasound.

• The operation of this device is the same as other portable ultrasounds and it is able to show images on a separate screen in color or black and white with high quality.

• This device does not need a wire to connect to the display and can be easily connected to it.

• The speed of viewing images on the screen with the help of this device is very high.

Complications and disadvantages of portable ultrasound

Ultrasound has been used for several years in all countries of the world as a safe and low-risk method to identify diseases and observe the internal organs of the body, and so far no special complications have been observed after its use. Because the portable ultrasound device works exactly like other ultrasound devices, so there is no expectation of complications and problems in this type of device.

In any case, it is possible that the heat and waves emitted by ultrasound devices may cause mild sensitivity for some people, although this is very rare. The heat transmitted by portable ultrasound is about 2 to 4 degrees Celsius, which Considering the physical conditions of people, it is very insignificant and cannot be dangerous for the human body in any way. But some patients may be sensitive to this.

For which people is it necessary to use portable ultrasound?

• The first group of people who need a portable ultrasound machine to perform ultrasound are pregnant mothers. Pregnant mothers, especially in the last months of pregnancy, have difficult conditions for mobility and movement. As a result, going to the doctor's office and sitting for hours for the ultrasound appointment is very annoying. The use of portable ultrasound means that there is no need to travel and stay in traffic or move a lot for the pregnant mother.

• The second group is people who have physical problems or heart problems. People who are unable to move, i.e. have spinal problems or arthritis, will have difficult conditions to move and use ultrasound services. For this reason, using portable ultrasound will be the best choice for them.

Also, people who suffer from cardiovascular problems, like many other people, if they want to use fixed ultrasound machines normally, they have to work for a long time from home until their turn arrives at the doctor's office, considering the conditions and crowding. It is very difficult and difficult.

• In addition, in some urgent cases that require early diagnosis, the doctor can use portable ultrasound for diagnosis so that less time is spent.

Types of ultrasound with the help of portable ultrasound

In medical science, there are several types of ultrasound, of which you may only be familiar with one or two. One of the types of ultrasound that almost everyone is familiar with is pregnancy ultrasound, which is performed to determine the age of the fetus and its health status. In the following, we introduce the types of ultrasound that can be performed using portable ultrasound:

• Mammogram

One of the types of ultrasound is called mammogram, which is performed to diagnose breast diseases and its condition. This ultrasound can be used to diagnose breast cancer and the presence of active lymph nodes and such.

• Radiography

Using portable ultrasound, even radiography is possible. The ultrasound machine uses sound waves. But radiography uses X-rays to observe the internal state of the body, the results of which are not shown on the screen. Rather, it should be placed separately on paper.

• Mobile ultrasound

Mobile ultrasound is used when the doctor intends to examine the state of movement, displacement and blood transfusion. This type of ultrasound can also be easily done at home. The resulting images are in color and will be displayed on the screen.

• Ultrasound of the heart

Heart echo can also be done using portable ultrasound. The process of echocardiography is exactly like an ultrasound and the results are recorded on paper. All these things can be done at home and the doctor can do it anywhere using portable ultrasound. (https://igg-med.com/)

Types of pregnancy ultrasound

In general, there are 2 important screening ultrasounds in pregnancy and all mothers should do:

1. Down syndrome screening

2. Ultrasound examination of fetal health

A routine ultrasound is done at two times during pregnancy.

1- Early pregnancy to see the heart and estimate the age of the fetus

2- during pregnancy for general examination of the fetus

First trimester pregnancy ultrasounds

1. Simple ultrasound: to assess the presence of the fetus and diagnose the gestational sac, the age of the fetus, check the fetal heart rate and hematoma in pregnancy

2. First screening ultrasound or NT ultrasound (NT-NB): The first important pregnancy ultrasound is performed at 11-14 weeks of pregnancy. Pay attention, the best time to do it is 12-13 weeks of pregnancy. In this ultrasound, which is also known as Down syndrome screening

nt and nb ultrasound have two basic and advanced types. In the ultrasound, the basic type of NT and NB is checked, and in the advanced type, in addition to these two variables, ductus venosus, tricuspid valve, IT and the number of umbilical cord vessels and in some cases the kidneys are also evaluated. (NT, NB, DV, TV, TVV)

Sifting is derived from the root of ghabil, which means sieve, and we use a sieve when we intend to separate. The purpose of screening for Down's syndrome is to separate suspected fetuses with the syndrome from healthy fetuses. It should be noted that there is always a possibility of error in screening because the goal is not diagnosis. The accuracy of Down syndrome screening is about 90%. In addition to ultrasound, a blood test is also performed in Down syndrome screening, which is also called NIPT, and its accuracy is about 98%, but this blood test is not usually performed.

If you are told that the fetus is suspicious in the first screening, diagnostic tests such as amniocentesis will be performed in the next step.

Second trimester pregnancy ultrasound

The second screening ultrasound or anomaly ultrasound is performed at the age of 18-19 weeks. The purpose of anomalous ultrasound is to check the health of the fetus and screen for fetal abnormalities from head to toe. In the ultrasound examination of the health of the fetus, in addition to examining all internal and external organs and organs of the fetus, the probability of contracting syndromes, including Down syndrome, is evaluated based on several markers. Legal abortion is not performed after the 19th week of pregnancy and the importance of this ultrasound is determined.

Echocardiography of the fetal heart

8 out of every 1000 fetuses have heart abnormalities, which shows the importance of heart examination. Fetal echocardiography is not performed for all people and is performed only in the following cases:

• High number of NT in the first screening

• History of heart disease in mother, father or previous children

Increased or decreased heart rate (tachycardia-bradycardia) or irregular heart rate (arrhythmia)

• There is a disturbance in examining the health of the fetus

• Vascular collagen rheumatological patients such as lupus or rheumatism: in these patients, there is a possibility of heart block in the fetus.

• Presence of pre-pregnancy diabetes in the mother

- The doctor suspects heart disorders

- Embryos from IVF

Doppler ultrasound of the fetus

In Doppler ultrasound, the blood flow of the fetus is examined based on the physical phenomenon called Doppler. Doppler ultrasound evaluates fetal blood circulation and oxygenation status, fetal oxygen deficiency (hypoxia), fetal response acidosis, arterial and venous disorders. If the fetal doppler is disturbed, the necessary measures should be taken in 48-72 hours. Also, as mentioned, another type of Doppler ultrasound is also performed along with NT ultrasound.

Third trimester pregnancy tests and ultrasounds

In the third trimester screening, the following are done:

Biophysical profile scoring: This ultrasound is performed along with fetal heart rate or NST. The purpose of doing it is to make a general evaluation in terms of the probability of fetal death and to estimate the probability of fetal death in order to decide on subsequent measures during childbirth.

Biometric ultrasound: examining the size of different parts of the fetus and the ratio of these sizes, which is effective in examining the health and growth of the fetus.

Types of common ultrasounds during pregnancy

The exact details of how to perform the ultrasound are slightly different, but usually the ultrasound is performed according to the same steps.

Two types of ultrasound are performed during pregnancy:

Abdominal ultrasound:

In this type of ultrasound, the doctor places a special gel on the pregnant woman's abdomen. After that, the ultrasound transducer () of the ultrasound machine can easily move on the gelled abdomen.

Vaginal ultrasound (Transvaginal ultrasound)

In vaginal ultrasound, a smaller ultrasound transducer is used. This transducer is inserted into the vagina and after that a more accurate and clear image of the internal space is obtained. Usually, this type of ultrasound is done in early pregnancy.

Does ultrasound during pregnancy have side effects?

Ultrasound has been used during pregnancy for more than 40 years, and no side effects from this method have been known so far. This method is completely safe and is necessary to ensure the normal development of the fetus in the mother's womb.

Reasons for the need for ultrasound during pregnancy

• Ultrasound is needed to ensure the correct implantation of the fertilized egg on the inner wall of the uterus and the formation of the placenta. Other reasons for the need for ultrasound include:

• To prevent ectopic pregnancy

• To prevent pregnancy complications such as molar (null) pregnancy and abortion

- To determine pregnancy

- To check the growth and development of the fetus

- To check birth defects and genetic abnormalities

- As part of other prenatal tests such as "placental villus sampling

How to perform pregnancy ultrasound

Ultrasound is a very simple method for imaging the fetus. After the mother lies down on the bed, the technician or radiologist applies a special gel to the abdomen and pelvis. This gel improves the connection between the uterus and the transducer so that the waves pass through the abdomen more correctly. After this, the device itself, which is the size of a palm, is placed on the abdomen. By moving the converter, black and white images can be seen on the monitor. The mother may be asked not to move or to hold her breath during the ultrasound.

Is ultrasound painful?

Under normal conditions, ultrasound does not hurt. However, if a person has a pelvic injury or abdominal pain, they may feel pain from the transducer pressure during the ultrasound.

Important points about ultrasounds during pregnancy Ultrasounds are necessary to check the health and growth of the fetus, therefore, you should not miss any of the predetermined ultrasounds.

Ultrasound should only be performed by a trained specialist or technician who has the ability to analyze the images.

If any abnormality is observed during the ultrasound, the doctor may use more methods and tests with higher resolution. Some parts of the body are difficult to distinguish during ultrasound, so the doctor can be asked to show them on the images. Ultrasound should not be painful under normal conditions, so in case of pain, the doctor should be informed immediately.

It is recommended that you wear comfortable, loose and suitable clothes for the ultrasound so that it is easier to access the abdomen.

You must drink plenty of water to prepare for the ultrasound. With this, the ultrasound will be done sooner and the images will have a higher resolution. Ultrasound during pregnancy is not only correct, but also effective. Ultrasound is also necessary to determine if you are pregnant or not. In case of pregnancy, ultrasound should be performed to check the stages of growth and development and the changes of the fetus properly. It is also important to consult your doctor regarding your health status during pregnancy.

What are 2D, 3D and 4D ultrasound?

Two-dimensional ultrasound is the most common and common type of ultrasound that is performed in black and white. 3D ultrasound is something similar to 4D, with the difference that a fixed image of the fetus is seen in it and it does not actually move. 4D ultrasound is a type of color ultrasound that shows the face of the fetus and its movements in 3 dimensions and the fourth dimension of the reactions of the fetus during a certain period of time. The mother can see reactions such as yawning, hiccups or thumb sucking in this ultrasound.

When should we do an ultrasound?

The Canadian Society of Obstetricians and Gynecologists recommends that all pregnant women have an ultrasound between the 18th and 22nd weeks of pregnancy.

Are 3D and 4D ultrasounds safe for mother and fetus?

When it comes to safety, there is really no difference between different ultrasounds. The same frequency is used in all ultrasounds. In the past 50 years of research, it has been shown that ultrasound does not pose any danger to the fetus, and in fact, ultrasound is one of the safest tools for examining the fetus and is accepted in almost all countries and in the medical systems of the world today.

What are the advantages of 3D and 4D ultrasounds?

These ultrasounds are performed to examine the fetus more closely. The results of the studies have shown that performing 3D and 4D ultrasounds indirectly increases the mother's maternal feelings and stimulating these maternal feelings makes them pay more attention to their nutrition or even to quit harmful habits during pregnancy such as smoking because they feel their child and confidently Since she is healthy, they will spend the pregnancy less anxious.

Can we always see a clear image of the fetus's face in 3D ultrasound?

Some 3D sono technologies and equipment allow you to see your baby's face clearly unless the fetus is in an unusual position, which can be due to the amount of fluid, the location of the placenta, and the way the hands are placed around the face. If the face is completely unclear, the ultrasound center is obliged to perform a repeat ultrasound for you without charging for it.

The best time to get 3D and 4D ultrasounds?

It depends on what you want to see. Many women like to do this twice during pregnancy, so if you belong to this group, we suggest one from the 20th to the 24th week and the other from the 26th to the 36th week. You will certainly see a more accurate picture of the fetus's face in the second ultrasound. In the first weeks, you will see more movement and movements, and in the later weeks, you will see a clearer picture of his face. After the 34th week, it becomes a little difficult to see a clear picture, but this is different for each fetus. The suggestion of the Canadian Society of Gynecologists is to do an ultrasound once between the 21st and 24th weeks.

Do you offer diagnostic ultrasounds? When?

This depends on the opinion of the doctor you are under, but it is usually suggested between the 18th and 22nd weeks.

How can we see a more accurate image in ultrasound?

Most experts suggest to increase your fluid intake to maintain health during pregnancy and especially before the ultrasound because drinking large amounts of water makes the amniotic fluid clear. The results of some studies have shown that if you drink a glass of natural juice half an hour before the 3D ultrasound, your fetus will be more alert during the ultrasound.

What is the duration of 3D and 4D sonos?

It usually takes between 15 and 30 minutes.

Can we do a 3D ultrasound but don't want to know the gender of our child?

it is possible. For some parents, not knowing the gender until the moment of birth is considered a surprise, so if you do not want to know the gender of your child, be sure to raise this issue before the ultrasound. (salamat.ir)

How is the ultrasound of children and babies?

Ultrasound is performed in children and infants for various reasons to diagnose their disease. For example, ultrasound may be done for children's constipation or ultrasound of newborns' kidneys. Whatever the reason, doing an ultrasound may seem a little worrying for parents, because they do not know exactly whether it is dangerous to use this method to definitively diagnose the type of illness of their child or not. Ultrasound is actually a safe and painless method that transmits images inside the body to the computer monitor through sound waves so that the doctor can examine the abdominal condition of the child or baby more carefully. For this purpose, a transducer called a probe is used to transfer the images to the monitor screen. Since these waves are ultrasound, there is no need to worry about the risk of radiation for the health of the child.

The use of ultrasound in children and infants in the diagnosis of diseases

Ultrasound is a painless method and is widely used today. Diagnostic ultrasound, also known as ultrasound, is an imaging method that uses high-frequency sound waves to produce images of body structures. These images can provide valuable information for the diagnosis and treatment of all kinds of diseases and physical conditions of the person. Ultrasound of children and babies is the same as the usual ultrasound, which can detect disorders inside the body by means of sound waves. With ultrasound, you can see internal organs, blood vessels and the structure of connective tissue. This imaging method is very useful for evaluating the causes of abdominal, pelvic, or scrotal pain in children. In general, ultrasound in children is similar to adults and does not differ much.

Application of ultrasound in children and babies

Children's ultrasound is done to check many different conditions and problems. Some of the common problems for which an ultrasound may be prescribed are:

• Appendicitis (inflammation of the appendix)

• Kidney or bladder stones

• Examining the testicles of the baby

• Who exists

• Abdominal abscess

Diagnosing reflux of bladder to urine and hydronephrosis (accumulation of urine in the kidney and increase in the size of the penis) in babies and infants

• As a guide for taking samples from the kidneys and other organs of the baby

• Kidney infections

• Acute pancreatitis

• Lymphadenopathy (lymphatic gland disease)

• Overgrown ovaries in female children.

• Soft tissue masses and protrusions

• Chronic abdominal pain

• Intussusception

Benefits of ultrasound for children and babies

1. Ultrasound is non-invasive (no needles or injections).

2. It doesn't hurt.

3. Ultrasound is widely used and cheaper than other imaging methods.

4. It is very safe and does not use radiation.

5. Ultrasound scan shows a clear image of soft tissues that are not well shown in X-ray images.

6. It is very useful for evaluating abdominal, pelvic or scrotal pain in children.

7. Standard diagnostic ultrasound has no known harmful effects on humans.

Special ultrasound for children

Pediatric ultrasound includes general and similar ultrasounds for adults as well as some specialized ultrasounds for children, which include the following in brief:

hip ultrasound

This specialized ultrasound is used to investigate the congenital dislocation of the pelvis. This ultrasound can often be done up to three months. In this ultrasound, certain angles in the baby's pelvis are measured, which can lead to the diagnosis of congenital dislocation of the hip. This ultrasound should be performed for all fetuses that are placed in a breech position; Because the risk of this disease is higher in fetuses that are breech.

Reflux ultrasound

In this ultrasound, the return of stomach acid to the esophagus in the baby is measured. To perform this ultrasound, the baby should be kept hungry for an hour and then breastfed during the ultrasound to determine the return of milk. Mothers who breastfeed their baby should express some of their milk and pour it into a bottle and feed the baby with a bottle during ultrasound.

Stomach pyloric ultrasound

In this ultrasound, the length and diameter of the stomach outlet are measured; Because one of the causes of frequent vomiting in babies is the narrowness of this outlet, which can be detected by ultrasound. To perform this ultrasound, the baby must be fed and the stomach must be completely full.

Procedures before ultrasound of children and infants

• Preparation of the child depends on the type of ultrasound. When planning your baby's ultrasound, ask the radiologist for dietary instructions before the procedure:

• The child should wear loose and comfortable clothes.

• The child may be asked to refrain from eating and drinking for a few hours before the ultrasound to better show the gallbladder and upper abdominal organs.

• The child is asked to drink several glasses of water and refrain from urinating an hour or two before the ultrasound. This causes the bladder to fill when the scan begins

Method of doing sonography of children and babies

During the ultrasound, the child should sit or lie on the bed, and it is better for the parents to stay with the child to help keep the child still, in addition to supporting him. Depending on the area of the body being scanned, your child may need to remove some clothing. A small amount of clear gel is poured over the area to be scanned and the ultrasound transducer is moved slowly across the body to be examined. Black, gray and white images appear on the screen and the sonographer saves all relevant images to be sent for interpretation.

Complications of ultrasound in children and infants

In general, newborn ultrasound is not harmful or dangerous; Because there are no X-rays in the radiation of the imaging device. Ultrasound does not cause any pain or harmful radiation for children.

Abdominal ultrasound in children

In abdominal ultrasound in children (children), sound waves are used to produce images of the inside of the body. It does not use radiation and has no known harmful effects. This method is very useful for evaluating the causes of abdominal, pelvic or scrotal pain in children.

Preparation for abdominal ultrasound in children depends on the type of exam. When scheduling your child's ultrasound, ask if there are any special instructions for eating and drinking before the exam. Your child should wear loose and comfortable clothes.

What is abdominal ultrasound imaging?

Ultrasound imaging is a non-invasive medical test that helps doctors diagnose and treat underlying diseases. It is safe and painless. It produces images of the inside of the body using sound waves. Ultrasound imaging is also called sonography. In this method, it uses a small probe called a transducer and a gel that is placed directly on the skin. High-frequency sound waves are transmitted from the probe through the gel to the body. The probe collects the sounds that come back.

The computer uses those sound waves to create an image. X-rays are not used in ultrasound examinations. Because ultrasound takes images in real time, it can show the structure and movement of the body's internal organs. These images can also show blood flow in blood vessels.

Pediatric abdominal ultrasound imaging produces images of the abdominal organs.

In some cases, the doctor may order Doppler ultrasound imaging along with an abdominal ultrasound to evaluate blood flow in certain abdominal arteries and veins.

How does abdominal ultrasound work?

Ultrasound imaging uses the same principles of sonar that bats, ships, and fishermen use. When a sound wave hits an object, it bounces back or echoes. By measuring these echo waves, it is possible to determine the distance of the object as well as its size, shape and consistency.

Doctors use ultrasound to detect changes in the appearance of organs, tissues and vessels and to detect abnormal masses such as tumors.

In an ultrasound examination, a transducer sends both sound waves and records the echo (return) waves. When the transducer is pressed against the skin, it sends small pulses of inaudible, high-frequency sound waves to the body. As sound waves bounce off organs, fluids, and internal tissues, a sensitive receptor in the transducer registers small changes in pitch and direction of the sound. A computer instantly measures these waves and displays them as images on a monitor. The technician usually captures one or more frames of moving images as still images. They may also store short video clips of images.

Doppler ultrasound, a special ultrasound technique, measures the direction and speed of blood cells as they move through the blood vessels. The movement of blood cells causes a change in the pitch of the reflected sound waves (called the Doppler effect). A computer collects and processes the sounds and creates graphs or color images that show the flow of blood in the blood vessels.

How is a children's abdominal ultrasound performed?

For most ultrasound exams, you lie face up on an exam table that can be tilted or moved. Patients may return to both sides to improve image quality.

The technician applies a clear, water-based gel to the area of the body being examined. This gel helps the transducer to communicate with the body better and more reliably. It is also effective in eliminating air pockets between the transducer and the skin. It even prevents sound waves from passing through your body. The technician or radiologist places the transducer on the skin in different places and examines the desired area. They may also angle the sound beam from another location to better see the target area.

Doctors perform Doppler ultrasound with the same transducer. When the exam is complete, the technician may ask you to get dressed and wait while he reviews the ultrasound images.

Ultrasound examination is usually completed within 30 minutes.

What will the child experience during and after the operation?

Most ultrasound examinations are painless, quick and easily tolerated. Your baby will lie face up on the examination table. The technician or radiologist may ask the patient to roll from side to side or maintain a prone position during part of the examination. The radiologist or technician spreads warm gel on the skin, then presses and moves the transducer firmly against the abdomen. The transducer moves back and forth to obtain the desired images. There may be slight pressure discomfort as the transducer is pressed against the area being examined.

If the area being scanned is sensitive, your child may feel pressure or slight pain. If a Doppler ultrasound study is performed, your baby may hear pulse-like sounds that change as blood flow is monitored and measured. After the examination, the gel is removed from your child's skin. After the test, children should be able to resume their normal activities.

A radiologist, a doctor trained to supervise and interpret radiology examinations, will analyze the images. The radiologist sends a signed report to the physician who requested the examination. Then the doctor will share the results with you. In some cases, the radiologist may share the results with you after the exam.

You may even need a follow-up examination so that the doctor can recheck the results of the treatment.

What are the limitations of abdominal ultrasound imaging?

Ultrasound waves are disturbed by air or gas. Therefore, ultrasound is not an ideal imaging technique for an air-filled bowel or organs covered by the bowel. Ultrasound is not useful for imaging air-filled lungs, but may be used to detect fluid around or within the lungs. Similarly, ultrasound cannot penetrate bone, but may be used to image a bone fracture or infection around the bone. Obese patients are more difficult to image with ultrasound because larger amounts of tissue weaken the sound waves as they pass through the body and must be returned to the transducer for analysis. (https://pezeshket.com/)

What measures are necessary to perform an ultrasound of animals?

Ultrasound is an examination that is requested as a complementary method for the diagnosis of many treatments and diseases. An experiment that does not have any complications and the only problem can be the animal's fear of new conditions. What points should we pay attention to before doing an ultrasound? By following what conditions can we be sure of accurate ultrasound results? Stay with us in this article so that while answering your important questions in this field, we will know how to prepare for animal ultrasound.

When do animals need ultrasound?

In the past few years, animal diseases have become very widespread. Despite the presence of various diseases, accurate diagnosis and treatment of diseases is not an easy task. In some cases, it is not possible to know the type of disease even from the external symptoms. To check the organs inside the animal's body, veterinarians request ultrasound. By using this method, various problems are diagnosed in the animal's body. If your animal has certain symptoms, the vet will prescribe an ultrasound. These symptoms can be one of the following:

• Abnormal weight loss

• Persistent diarrhea and vomiting

• The presence of internal infections, especially infections related to the uterus

•   Frequent urination

• Pregnancy and reproduction

How is animal ultrasound performed?

Ultrasound is a simple and painless test. Although this does not cause any concern, being in a new situation may make the animal afraid. When the animal does not know what action is going to be done on him, he unconsciously gets stressed. Add this situation to a situation where the animal is restless and in pain due to its illness. In this situation, the vet will most likely inject your little friend with a sedative.

Preliminary preparations before ultrasound

When the examination does not work to find out the animal's disease, the veterinarian will ask you to perform various tests. Ultrasound is also a way to diagnose diseases that is done through high-frequency sound waves. If ultrasound is the way to diagnose the disease, how should we prepare our animal before doing it? In the rest of the article, we will answer this important question.

Shave the animal's belly hair

One of the most challenging things that occurs during ultrasound is shaving the hair of the abdomen. A topic that can be unpleasant for the owner of the animal. Losing part of body hair has a negative effect on the beauty of animals. Anyway, to get an accurate result, there is no other way than to remove a part of the animal's body hair. Since ultrasound requires direct contact with the skin, any obstructions must be removed from the skin. These obstacles can be body hair, skin lesions or dirt in the desired area. These obstacles are removed by the veterinarian to obtain accurate results before the ultrasound.

Fasting

Another important issue that is often overlooked is the fact that the animal is fasting or consuming heavy food. We recommend that you avoid giving your pet bulky and solid foods 6 to 8 hours before the ultrasound. Digestive activities begin in the stomach and intestines with the consumption of food. An event that causes a large volume of gas in the digestive system. Naturally, in this situation, we cannot have a complete and accurate examination of the animal's body. Due to this important issue, avoid giving food to animals before going to veterinary clinics or hospitals.

Water and liquid consumption

Consuming water and liquids does not cause problems for ultrasound. Consumption of liquids is not only prohibited, but also facilitates the work process. Because drinking water helps to produce urine. A veterinarian who is looking for an ultrasound of organs such as kidneys or bladder will definitely ask you to give your animal water for a better diagnosis. Therefore, make sure that the animal does not urinate before the test.

Does the ultrasound need to be repeated?

One of the important questions that arise in relation to animal ultrasound is the number of times it is repeated. During the pregnancy of pets, ultrasound may be performed several times. The veterinarian will ask you to take several ultrasounds to ensure the health of the mother animal and her fetus. Sometimes, according to the veterinarian's diagnosis, ultrasound is performed periodically.

If your pet has had surgery, the vet may order another ultrasound. In some cases, because the ultrasound results are not accurate, it needs to be repeated. For example, when the animal's bladder is not full, the veterinarian asks you to visit the clinic at another time for an ultrasound. In general, according to the veterinarian's diagnosis and the type of disease the animal is suffering from, the number of times of ultrasound varies.

Refer to reputable clinics

Ultrasound of animals, just like ultrasound of human organs, requires expertise and skill. We recommend that you get your pets ultrasound done by or under their supervision. Let's not forget that the more powerful the ultrasound device is, the more accurate the result will be. On the other hand, the use of such devices leads to the high cost of ultrasound.

Another important issue that you need to pay attention to is visiting specialized centers and reputable clinics. Considering the time and money you spend on your pet's treatment, pay attention to these important things when performing an ultrasound.

Care after ultrasound

After you have done your pet's ultrasound, wait for the results. Ultrasound does not cause any problems for animals and you can leave the animal at home as usual. Meanwhile, some people are worried about the complications of ultrasound. You need to know that ultrasound does not cause any side effects.

What is a veterinary ultrasound machine?

Since the early 1980s, ultrasound has been considered a unique procedure in veterinary medicine. The use of ultrasound to check the condition of sick animals and livestock diseases is increasing day by day.

Fixed ultrasound machines or portable ultrasound machines are used in veterinary hospitals in big cities. In the last decade, the use of portable ultrasound devices has gradually become common in veterinary clinical diagnosis.

Veterinary ultrasound machine is one of the important equipment in veterinary medicine and a great advantage for veterinarians. Considering that the animal is not able to describe its history and declare its illness, the veterinarian needs a picture of the internal space of the animal's body to know the problems and start the treatment. With ultrasound devices, the veterinarian will be able to image the inside of the body of animals such as cows, sheep, horses, goats, dogs and cats.

Veterinary ultrasound, commonly used to diagnose diseases, is a device that uses ultrasound waves, or ultrasonic waves, with a frequency of 1.5 to 15 MHz. These rays are completely safe and can be used repeatedly and at different times to diagnose small animal diseases and provide appropriate images of the animal's body. Of course, having an ultrasound done on a pet can be a bit uncomfortable, but a mild sedative can be used to calm the patient down.

The best veterinary ultrasound machine

What is the best veterinary ultrasound machine and which country is it made in? The answer to the question is a bit difficult because it completely depends on the need and the amount of budget you have considered for the purchase of a pet ultrasound machine.

Today, you can buy an ultrasound machine at a much lower cost than in the past, but before buying a veterinary ultrasound machine, answer the following questions to make the best choice when buying an ultrasound machine for animals.

What kind of animals do you do ultrasound?

The answer to this question is very important. If you are scanning light animals or animals such as dogs or cats, there is a light animal ultrasound machine, and if you are scanning heavy animals such as horses and cows, there is a heavy animal ultrasound machine.

Heavy livestock ultrasound system

For the ultrasound of heavy animals, you need a portable ultrasound device and it is very important that this device has a high penetration depth because the heavy animal is large and the penetration depth of the probe of your ultrasonic device and the frequency of your probe should be higher

Also, in the ultrasound of heavy cows, you need linear endorectal probes to be able to perform better scans. Of course, your Kanox probe must also have a suitable penetration depth, which depends a lot on the type and frequency you choose when buying a livestock ultrasound scanner.

The next thing to pay attention to when buying a heavy livestock ultrasonic device is that the more durable the device and its body is resistant to impact and water penetration, the more suitable this ultrasound unit is for your work.

Light livestock ultrasound machine

Veterinary ultrasound for low weight and small animals has become much more practical today and is used in most veterinary clinics.

Usually, pet ultrasound scanners are of the portable type, which takes up less space and is easy to move, but sometimes the treatment center prefers to get a very different furnished device. In fact, mobile devices are more durable than handheld devices and also have more processing power.

Of course, there is a portable veterinary ultrasound machine that is of very high quality and can compete with the supplied ultrasound machine, but in veterinary centers it is recommended to use portable ultrasound machines because they are easy to move and maneuver more information offers

Ultrasound machine components

This device consists of the following parts:

- Power supply

- Special display for displaying measured information

• Canox, linear and transvaginal types of probes. The linear probe is used for surface surveys with less depth. While the Kanox probe is intended for detection in deeper tissues.

Livestock ultrasound should have high imaging accuracy and not produce sound. It is also necessary that the created image be uniform and clearly show different parts of the texture. It should be noted that sonographic skill is effective in creating the right image because it must be able to place the probe of the device in the best position and the best angle to see the inside of the patient's body well.

The images produced by the ultrasound system are usually black and white, but in more advanced models, color and 3 or 4 dimensional images are also displayed. Although there are imaging methods with better quality than ultrasound, this method is less expensive and less dangerous for the animal and is completely non-invasive.

Veterinary ultrasound device applications

Animal ultrasound devices for applications such as pregnancy diagnosis, gender determination, twinning, ovarian disorders, uterine disorders, early pregnancy detection in cows and horses, diagnosis of cancerous cysts and ovarian tumors, uterine infections, prevention, treatment and control of metabolic diseases. Such as ketosis, fatty liver, hypocalcemia, management of non-pregnant cows, evaluation of the herd for breeding status, management of buying and selling livestock.

Types of veterinary ultrasound devices

• Furnished ultrasound machine

Furnished ultrasound machines are equipped with a keyboard, a large monitor and a console. These devices are used for specialized imaging in veterinary clinics. These devices are not portable due to their size, dimensions and weight. Therefore, the purchase of these devices is not recommended for use in veterinary medicine due to the very high price.

The use of the provided ultrasound device is recommended for clinics that often perform dog and cat ultrasound. The price of these ultrasonic devices is very high.

• Portable ultrasound device

Portable ultrasound machines weigh less than standard ultrasound machines, so they are easier to transport. Some portable devices are the size of a laptop and may or may not have a battery. A group of portable ultrasound devices are very light and small, which are called portable.

• Handheld portable ultrasound device

Handheld portable ultrasound machines weigh about 400 to 600 grams and are known as ultra-small portable ultrasound machines, portable ultrasound machines, pocket ultrasound machines, and personal ultrasound machines. These devices fit in the pocket like a mobile phone. Portable ultrasound machines are compact and battery operated. Handheld ultrasound devices are considered suitable for examining light and heavy livestock.

Factors affecting the price of veterinary ultrasound equipment

• Device brand

• Number of probes and accessories

- The technology used in making the device

- User designed for imaging

- Hardware and software features and facilities

Tips for buying a veterinary ultrasound machine

Veterinary ultrasound devices are marketed for diagnostic purposes and are not intended for treatment. The probe is one of the main components of the animal ultrasound system. The ultrasound probe creates an image of the animal's body by sending ultrasound waves to the animal's body and receiving their return wave. These waves are converted into images by the very powerful processor of the device, which can be seen on the screen or monitor of the ultrasound scanner.

Therefore, one of the criteria that should be considered when buying a veterinary ultrasound machine is the probe of the machine and the frequency covered by it. Each probe works with a specific frequency. Therefore, the accuracy of animal ultrasound equipment depends on various parameters. These parameters can have a direct impact on the purchase or sale of veterinary ultrasound equipment. Veterinarians should note that there is no need to spend a lot of money when buying a cow or sheep ultrasound machine. A high price of a pet ultrasound machine does not necessarily mean that it is better for the user.

What are the features of the ultrasound center?

Features of the ultrasound center: You may need an ultrasound for various reasons, but in all these cases, choosing a reliable ultrasound center is a separate issue that affects the results. It is obvious that the skill of performing ultrasound is effective and this diagnostic method can lead to completely correct or distorted diagnosis.

For this reason, it is necessary to choose an ultrasound center with the utmost care and attention and to perform this diagnostic method in a reliable place.

1. Choose an ultrasound center that has sufficient accreditation and experience.

Many centers in cities provide these services, of course, except for cases of violation, all of them have the necessary licenses. However, to get the best result, we recommend that you go to a reputable and experienced center.

This makes the result of your ultrasound completely reliable and if there is or is not a problem in it, you can follow the next medical decisions with confidence.

In many cases, delay in diagnosis or wrong diagnosis has irreparable consequences for people.

2. Pay attention to the level of cleanliness and hygiene in this center.

Not only these days, when the world community is involved with the corona virus, but also you should always pay attention to the level of cleanliness and hygiene in medical and diagnostic centers.

This is a predetermined protocol for these centers and unfortunately it is sometimes ignored.

Therefore, be careful enough to see if the center you are looking for is at level one in terms of hygiene and its principles.

3. Check the time allotted for each ultrasound scan.

In some ultrasound or radiography centers, the work routine has taken on a commercial form, and in order to accept more patients and clients in one working day, little time is taken to perform each ultrasound, and the detection rate is low.

For this reason, it is necessary to be careful that the matters related to ultrasound and diagnosis are done completely calmly and without haste, and enough time is allocated for each patient and client.

4. Note that the ultrasound center you are looking for has all the services.

These services include:

- sonography
- Mammography
- Breast elastography
- Breast sampling
- Thyroid sampling
- Mammography of breasts with prosthesis
- Radiography
- Wiring
- Galactograph

for you. If the center you are looking for is not fully equipped and does not provide full services, you will have to go to other centers for some additional diagnostic methods, and this procedure will disrupt your diagnosis and treatment.

resources

1- Comparison of fetal weight estimation with clinical method, ultrasound and the combined formula of ultrasound and mother's weight - Authors:

Shahla Yazdani Bouzari Zaint al-Sadat Elah Nazari Maliha Bijani Ali

Publication: Iran Midwifery and Infertility Journal - Year: 2013

2- Ultrasound device from components to application from the engineering and medical point of view

Authors: Alborzi Kasri Albarzi Kia Sanaz Iranshahi Ahmad Mehroz shrine Saharanord Saeed Abdullahzadeh Hossein - year 2013

3- Diagnostic value of ultrasound in biliary atresia

Authors: Rafii Mandana Nemati Masoud Nazarpour Samad

Publication: Medical Journal of Tabriz University of Medical Sciences

Year: 1388

4- Accuracy of ultrasound by the surgeon in non-penetrating abdominal trauma

Authors: Khosh Mohabbate Hadi Panahi Farzad Mehrovaz Shaaban | Mohibi Hasan Ali Baqarpour Jahormi Ali -- Publication: Kausar Medical Journal -- Year: 1389

5- Comparison of three diagnostic methods for determining gestational age with ultrasound

Authors: Nazanin Farshchian Iran Far Shirin | Rezaei Mansour

Publication: Journal of Kermanshah University of Medical Sciences (Bahboud)

Year: 1386

6- Ultrasound and radiology clinic site

7- Pajhwok (https://pezhvaksono.ir/blog/sonography/)

8- Pars imaging center:

https://parsimaging.ir/articles/%D8%B3%D9%88%D9%86%D9%88%DA%AF%D8%B1%D8%A7%D9%81%DB%8C-%D8%AF%D8%A7%D9%BE%D9%84%D8%B1-%D8%B1%D9%86%DA%AF%DB%8C-%DA%86%DB%8C%D8%B3%D8% AA-%D9%88-%DA%86%D9%87-%DA%A9%D8%A7%D8%B1%D8%A8%D8%B1%D8%AF%D9%87/)

9-https://soroush-sonography.ir/%D8%B3%D9%88%D9%86%D9%88%DA%AF%D8%B1%D8%A7%D9%81%DB%8C-% DA%86%D9%87%D8%A7%D8%B1-%D8%A8%D8%B9%D8%AF%DB%8C/

10-https://www.radiologymarkazi.ir/

11- https://irandamparvar.ir/%D8%AF%D8%B3%D8%AA%DA%AF%D8%A7%D9%87-%D8%B3%D9%88%D9%86%D9%88%DA%AF%D8%B1%D8%A7%D9%81%DB%8C-%D8%AF%D8%A7%D9%85%D9%BE%D8%B2%D8%B4%DA%A9%DB%8C-%DA%86%DB%8C%D8%B3%D8%AA/

12-https://nabipour-dr.com/%D8%A7%D8%B2-%D8%AA%D8%A7%D8%B1%DB%8C%D8%AE%DA%86%D9%87-%D8%B3%D9%88%D9%86%D9%88%DA%AF%D8%B1%D8%A7%D9%81%DB%8C-%DA%86%D9%87-%D9%85 %DB%8C%E2%80%8C-%D8%AF%D8%A7%D9%86%DB%8C%D8%AF%D8%9F/

1-<u>Pediatric Ultrasound, Part 2, An Issue of Ultrasound Clinics, Volume 5-1</u>

Books

- **Edition** 1st
- **Author** Brian D. Coley
- **Published** 22nd April 2010

2-<u>Musculoskeletal Ultrasound, An Issue of Ultrasound Clinics, Volume 7-3</u>

Books

- **Edition** 1st
- **Author** Diana Gaitini
- **Published** 8th October 2012

3-<u>Ultrasound in Medicine & Biology</u>

Journals

- **Volume** 1
- **ISSN** 0301-5629
- Journal website

4-<u>Ultrasound-Guided Procedures, An Issue of Ultrasound Clinics, Volume 4-1</u>

Books

- **Edition** 1st

- **Author** Hisham Tchelepi
- **Published** 21st August 2009

5-<u>Ultrasound, An Issue of Radiologic Clinics of North America, Volume 57-3</u>

Books

- **Edition** 1st
- **Author** Jason M. Wagner
- **Published** 29th March 2019

6-<u>Adaptive time gain compensation for ultrasonic imaging</u>

Ultrasound Med. Biol.

(1992)

- F. Destrempes *et al.*

7-<u>A critical review and uniformized representation of statistical distributions modeling the ultrasound echo envelope</u>

UltraSound Med. Biol.

(2010)

- D. Napolitano

8-<u>Sound speed correction in ultrasound imaging</u>

Ultrasonics

(2006)

- C. Yoon *et al.*

9-<u>In vitro estimation of mean sound speed based on minimum average phase variance in medical ultrasound imaging</u>

Ultrasonics

(2011)

- M. Maggioni *et al.*

10-<u>Optimization techniques for sparse matrix–vector multiplication on GPUs</u>

J. Parallel Distrib. Comput.

(2016)

- R.E. Zubajlo

11-<u>Experimental validation of longitudinal speed of sound estimates in the diagnosis of hepatic steatosis (part II)</u>

12-Ultrasound Med. Biol.

(2018)

- R. E. McKeighen and M. P. Buchin, "New techniques for dynamically variable electronic delays for real time ultrasonic...
- R.J. Mailloux

13-Phased array theory and technology

Proc. IEEE

(1982)

- H.T. Friis *et al.*

14-A multiple unit steerable antenna for short-wave reception

Proc. Inst. Radio Eng.

(1937)

- P.J. Kahrilas

15-HAPDAR—An operational phased array radar

Proc. IEEE

(1968)

16- Coupling myocardium and vortex dynamics in diverging-wave echocardiography

IEEE Trans Ultrason Ferroelectr Freq Control

(2019)

17-The effect of dynamic range alterations in the estimation of contrast

18-IEEE Trans. Ultrason. Ferroelectr. Freq. Control

(2019)

18-Experimental evaluation of spectral-based quantitative ultrasound imaging using plane wave compounding

19-IEEE Trans. Ultrason. Ferroelectr. Freq. Control

(Nov. 2014)

20-https://www.radiologyinfo.org/en/info/genus

21-https://www.radiologyinfo.org/en/info/abdomus-pdi

writers

Farshid Aramjoo	Mahdi kolahdouz ghouchani
aramjoofarshid@gmail.com	mahdikolahdouzghouchani@gmail.com

contact us

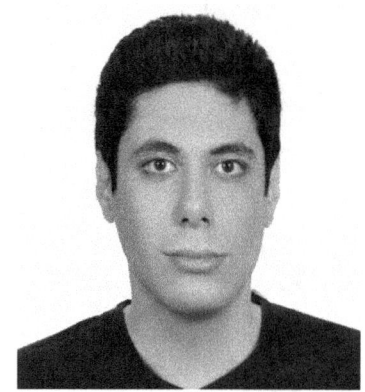 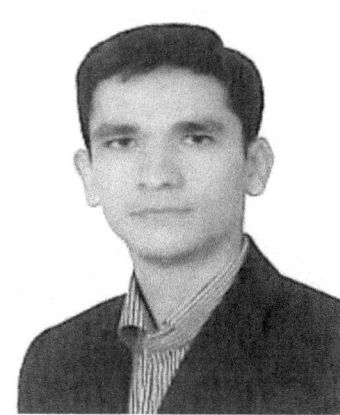

www.ingramcontent.com/pod-product-compliance
Lightning Source LLC
Chambersburg PA
CBHW062120220526
45471CB00010B/3815